Don't Touch My Foley!

A Book of Experiences and Lessons for Nurses and Healthcare Workers

by

Marilyn A. Lewis, MS, RN.

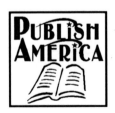

PublishAmerica
Baltimore

© 2010 by Marilyn A. Lewis, MS, RN.
All rights reserved. No part of this book may be reproduced, stored in a retrieval system or transmitted in any form or by any means without the prior written permission of the publishers, except by a reviewer who may quote brief passages in a review to be printed in a newspaper, magazine or journal.

First printing

PublishAmerica has allowed this work to remain exactly as the author intended, verbatim, without editorial input.

ISBN: 978-1-61546-740-2
PUBLISHED BY PUBLISHAMERICA, LLLP
www.publishamerica.com
Baltimore

Printed in the United States of America

Preface

As a nurse of 20 plus years, I was always there for my patients; gave 100% of my efforts to performing with the right intention and left work (most of the time) feeling I did a worthwhile job. Nursing has made me what I am: a person and fellow human being with patience, compassion, and understanding. In January, 2004, my entire perspective was to change when I became a critical care patient for the first time. I learned more about my patients as a ***patient***. I hope that what I share in this book helps healthcare workers re-examine their approach and perspectives to patient care.

Acknowledgments

This book wouldn't have been a reality without the wonderful doctors and nurses who worked so hard to keep me alive during the severe condition I was in. The nurses in the unit, stood by my side, caring for me, talking to me and holding my hand when I needed it. My husband, Gail was at my side every moment, stroking my hair and whispering words of love and encouragement. My dear daughter, Annette, was my cheerleader, stepping up to the "plate" and making sure my needs were being met. I won't mention names, but my supervisor was at my side every moment, calling the priest when I needed him, "as all good Catholics girls do!" we would say so often. I give her most sincere thanks.

And to anyone else I failed to remember; you know who you are. To you and everyone,

Thank you!

Chapter 1: The Beginning

I entered nursing school in 1982 while living in Kentucky with my husband, Gail and daughter, Annette, age 9. We lived on a 2300 acre farm with house, chicken coups and plenty of room to plant a garden. I was given a lay-off notice from my job as a nursing assistant at the local hospital, so I was free to stay at home and focus on my studies.

The two years in school were difficult. My husband worked as a farm hand on a local tobacco farm. He would leave at the crack of dawn and, along with 10 other farm hands, toil the tobacco fields until dusk. He would come home and continue to work in our garden until bedtime. We didn't have a phone so I would drive to the nearest carry-out and use the pay phone to call my mother or other family members. We had a cistern, a type of well on the property that had a leak, so as a result, we had my husband's boss bring in a tank of water hauled on a truck every 2-3 weeks. At times, I would stack up dirty dishes until they were all used up before washing them or, share my bath with my little daughter in order to save on water.

Because our income was so limited, we had to be resourceful and literally "live off the land." Each spring, we planted a large vegetable garden. Later in the fall, I would can or freeze our harvest, saving many trips to the grocery. I had a large pantry for storing canning jars and a large vented box for placing potatoes so they could last all winter. As for meat, Gail would go out into the woods and shoot, squirrel, rabbit, quail and pheasant. Upon his return, he would skin his kill and soak it in a brine to eliminate the "wild" taste in the meat. We were never hungry and actually, fried rabbit and squirrel are quite good with pan gravy!

The house we lived in had 25 rooms. We closed the upstairs and basically used the space down below. Now, I'm not talking about a home with all the finest of modern decor or appliances. This was a 100+ year old farmhouse with huge rooms and high ceilings. The water and electricity were installed 20 years earlier. We had to depend on wood-burning stoves for warmth during the winter months or use a fireplace. Being resourceful, my husband, Gail, would gather wood during warm months for "seasoning" and use the wood for burning in the stove when it got cold. In the spring and summer, it did get quite hot, so I would open the windows on the east and west ends of the house. A wonderful breeze would flow through bringing with it the scent of honeysuckle that grew at the side of the house. Many an evening, I would pile my nursing books on my bed and after hours of study, fall asleep to the scent of that honeysuckle in the room.

While I attended school, I still had to make sure I was meeting the needs of our daughter, Annette. At the time I entered school, she was 9 years old. Very precocious, Annette had already developed a sense of responsibility. She was an only child and learned early to pick up in her room, put away her toys and help out with the housework. We had a chicken coup with no chickens, so instead, Annette was allowed to have cats. By the time I graduated, she had 10 cats, each with a name and loving them as her own.

Christmas was a difficult time for us. We had little income and anything spent beyond basic needs was too much. As it was, my husband was earning minimum wages as a farm hand and during the winter, the work was minimal. I was collecting unemployment. I remember wrapping 2 Christmas presents one year for Annette. I'll never forget her getting up excited with anticipation only to find the 2 presents under the tree. She looked up at us and said, "Wasn't I good all year?"

Our hearts were broken! How do you answer a question like that? "Of course you have been good!" I said. We sat down and explained the situation as simply as possible. Annette listened with tears in her eyes. I promised her that if she would continue to help me as she was doing, and was patient until I could graduate, she would get everything on her Christmas list. The year I graduated, I had Annette make out the list of presents she would like to find under the tree. We spent Christmas in Michigan with my Mother that year, so Gail and I brought 30 presents to place under Mom's tree. Christmas morning found Annette up at 5 am, running down the stairs to see what she could find. The look on her face was priceless! Her big, blue eyes widened like saucers as she found every package she picked up had her name on it. After everyone finished unwrapping their gifts, Annette realized something. She then said, "Mommy, you got all the gifts on my list!" I told her we did indeed because she was worth it and deserved them. This was one Christmas I will remember for a long time.

During the last 6 months of my second year of nursing school, my husband and a friend of ours, started an airfreight business in Ohio. The job essentially took Gail all over the country delivering items that could only be shipped per ground transportation. There were times he was gone 1-2 weeks which became very lonely and overwhelming for Annette and me. We managed though, making frequent trips to the pay phone just to hear Gail's voice. Fortunately, I was coming to the end of my final semester and looking forward to all of us being together as a family again.

My Nursing Pinning Ceremony and Graduation were beautiful. Gail, Annette and I were not only excited about my graduating, but we were to embark on a new "journey" as we moved to Ohio the day after graduation. Family members came over to help us pack and we moved to Troy, Ohio, a lovely city just north of Dayton. We stayed temporarily with Gail's brother, Lonnie, and his wife, Gerry. They made us feel welcome and I was ready to start my career as a new graduate nurse! Several months later, I received a letter from the Ohio State Board of Nursing congratulating me on passing my nursing exam for licensure. I stared at the letter in disbelief; after the years of sacrifice on my part and that of my husband and daughter, I could now proudly declare I was a REGISTERED NURSE!

The years we lived in Kentucky were difficult, but I have such wonderful memories of how the three of us pulled together so I could finish school. We lived on approximately $10,000 year during the time I was in school. We had only what we absolutely needed, but we were happy and knew our situation would get better in time. Occasionally, we will take a drive up into Kentucky and visit that old farm. The house we lived in has since been torn down. The 100 foot driveway is still there and you can see the honeysuckle vines growing against the fence, reminding me of how many nights the scent of that delicate flower got me through hours of study.

To anyone reading this book, I feel it necessary to share this part of my personal life so that you can understand that I take my profession very seriously. Not only did I work feverishly to get through school, but my husband and daughter shared in the work as well. It was a team effort for us as Nursing is in general. You cannot be a good nurse if you are not a team member. My belief is that if I failed in my duty to finish school, I fail my husband and daughter too. My goal was anything BUT that. Starting with Chapter 2, you will find at the end "Points to Ponder." When I discuss a certain aspect of nursing care, I will describe my experience and then, apply the points to ponder or reflect on at the end of the chapters.

Chapter 2: Illness

I find it difficult to discuss this part of my book because it brings back many painful memories in my life. You need to understand that what I am about to explain is complicated in medical terminology, so I am going to use some lay terms so everyone can interpret what is said.

When I was 29 years old, (6 years prior to my nursing graduation), I was diagnosed with Cushing's Syndrome, an endocrine disorder affecting the adrenal glands. For those of you who are students, the endocrine system consists of organs whose primary function is in the metabolism of different parts of the body. The adrenal glands, lie on the kidneys and work at controlling fluid and electrolyte balance, heart rate, your "flight or fight"/ stress management and hormonal functions of other organs. You can look in your biology books to get a better explanation.

In my situation, the adrenals were enlarged and both had benign tumors requiring removal. I had all the classic symptoms of Cushing's and my doctor was instrumental in getting me the best help at the time. Dr. Robinson was an instructor of Wright State Medical School in Dayton, Ohio. Because of his training, he was able to recognize the symptoms, get me into the hospital and find the right surgeon to operate. I owe him my life. I also owe Dr. David Westbrock, the endocrinologist, for explaining the complexity of the disease I was about to face and reinforce to me the seriousness of taking my medications and making sure other doctors understood my condition. The bilateral adrenalectomy was successful. I was in the hospital for approximately 6 days after which, spent several difficult months at home recovering and adjusting to the changes occurring in my body. Dr. Westbrock explained to me that once my adrenals were removed, I would no longer have Cushing's but, instead, Addison's Disease. Sometimes known as adrenal-insufficiency, Addison's requires daily replacement doses of steroids. Some patients with Addison's still have their adrenal glands, but the glands are not functioning up to par. Such an example is President John F. Kennedy. He had Addison's Disease with the adrenal glands. He received daily injections of steroids so his body could function properly. In my case, both adrenals were removed. I have to take steroids daily TO LIVE! The steroids replace what my adrenals would have produced. OK. The following is the most important lesson to remember. ***Anyone with Addison's has to take steroids daily in order for their body to function properly***. The blood pressure, fluid/electrolyte balance and daily stressors are managed by the steroids. In my case, the steroids are keeping me alive, ***LITERALLY***! Should I forget a dose, run out of my steroids, I will go into an Addisonian Crisis which can begin with signs and symptoms of heart failure, leading to death. Another lesson to remember is that those patients with Addison's have a difficult time handling any kind of stress be it from illness, emotional upsets and yes, even exciting or positive stressors in life. During my lifetime since receiving the diagnosis of Addison's Disease, I have faced situations when I was hospitalized with asthma problems or had surgeries of various kinds. Each event required "stress doses" of steroids administered IV/IM.

Had I not been given the steroids, I would have gone into heart failure and/or faced death. The steroids assist my organs handle the stress overload of illness. In cases when I was to fly to Michigan to visit my Mother, the excitement and anticipation required my having to take a "stress dose" of steroids. This is the story of my life for the past 30 years. At this stage of my life, I am experiencing chronic pain in my back, legs and feet. If the pain gets out of hand, I have to take a "stress dose" of steroids to avoid heart failure. Naturally, steroids in themselves produce problems. Look in any drug manual and you can find all the side effects of steroids including elevated blood sugar, fluid retention, weight gain, etc. Not a nice drug, but I'll take it when it saves my life.

Points to Ponder

1. When assigned to a patient, review their diagnosis and medications related to their disease process. Review the doses, side effects and administration times of the medications.

2. Discuss with the patient their disease process. Find out how much the patient knows about their disease, the medications and if they have been compliant in taking their medications.

3. Monitor medications. Watch for any problems that may exist regarding possible synergistic or adverse effects of medications taken by the patient.

4. Medications such as steroids can cause a rise in blood sugar which necessitates the need for blood sugar monitors every shift or as ordered by the physician.

5. **Listen to your patients complaints**. They know what they are feeling. Make sure you monitor their level of pain from 0-10.

6. Monitor for any change in mental status, speech, mobility and behaviors. Report any of these changes to the attending physician. Keep in mind that medications can directly affect a patient's mood and mental status.

7. Provide emotional support for the patient. Listen and be empathetic of their feelings and what they may be going through besides their hospitalization.

8. Include support of surrounding family members. Include the family in the patient's plan of care as long as the patient permits.

Chapter 3: Career Focused

After graduation, Gail, Annette and I stayed in Ohio 10 years. My nursing career was on target and I set particular goals for myself. I started out working as a nursing supervisor for a 150 bed long-term care facility. I really enjoyed working with the elderly. They helped me to see how fragile life is and that I don't have to be afraid of getting old. Several years later, I was hired at one of the local hospitals as staff nurse on a medical floor. I was occasionally sent to the Pediatric unit. During this period of time, I became ill with a full-blown bowel obstruction. I had surgery; a colon resection and eventually recuperated and went back to work. Our father had diverticulitis and had to have a colostomy. He eventually died at the age of 56 as a result of complications. Unfortunately, our Father passed on the weak gene of bowel problems to each of us children. To date, we have all experienced surgery of one kind or another on our colons. This includes my two younger sisters, our brother and me.

Illness didn't stop me from pursuing my dreams as a nurse. I eventually went on to become an Assistant Director then, a Director of Nursing for a 200 bed skilled Nursing facility. I did well, passing several Department of Health surveys. This position was short lived because I eventually witnessed unethical practices of an administrator, and decided to resign. I told the Regional Administrator of the company I worked for that unethical practices were taking place. The company didn't investigate the information I gave them and so, the practices continued. Six months later after resigning,, I received a phone call from the Regional Administrator who informed me that the company eventually found out of the "practices" occurring at the nursing facility. He apologized for the company, stating that they would like me to come back as the Director. As much as liked this Administrator, I laughed and said I couldn't come back to a company that didn't believe me in the first place! He stated he understood perfectly and wished me luck in my future endeavors. I did the same. Last time I heard, that unscrupulous administrator was eventually fired, and works as a janitor in a nursing home somewhere in Ohio. So much for justice!

The next couple of years brought me much satisfaction and the realization that I actually found my "niche" in Nursing. I was hired at a free-standing psychiatric hospital. I worked on a dual-diagnosis unit, meaning we had patients in alcohol and drug detox as well as psychiatric patients. I found that this work was right up my alley. You just don't go into this type of nursing without some kind of personal attachment to it. In other words, I had some issues regarding co-dependency and alcoholism. I was the eldest of 5 children and remember vividly holding pillows over my head so I couldn't hear our Dad cursing at our Mother at 2:30 AM. I grew up with the fear of Daddy walking into the house on a Saturday afternoon while my friends were visiting me. He had done this before and humiliated me with his loud and boisterous voice. It's funny when I think about this, but when he was sober, Daddy was a wonderful man. He was comical, played with us and was a very friendly in general until he started to drink. Once I got into adulthood, I was able to move away from home and the craziness. Daddy died in January of 1977. It was a sad time but I know for our Mother, it was also a time of peace and relief for her.

I stayed at the psychiatric hospital approximately 5 years. I made some great friends, especially Barbara. She and her husband, Gene, decided to move to Tennessee because Gene was retiring from GM due to a cardiac ailment. Gail and I started to come down to Tennessee to visit Barb and Gene on a regular basis over a period of a couple of years. As we ended each visit, Gail and I developed a fondness for the area just North of Knoxville. I remember crying, not wanting to leave at all! In early Spring of 1994, Gail and I decided to make the move to Tennessee. My job in Ohio was in jeopardy. The hospital was downsizing and there was talk of lay-off. I had an opportunity to get a job where Barbara worked. The hospital was in the area, and I could get a full-time job right away. I sent in my resume' and in no time, I was heading to Tennessee for several interviews. I was hired that very day and started working July 11, 1994. I started out as a floor nurse, but eventually was promoted to Assistant Manager for 2 units on night shift. I also assisted the house supervisors whenever they were tied up. I eventually became a house supervisor on day shift for 6 months. Then it happened! I applied for the position of Manager for the Psychiatric unit in 2002. I was so excited when my supervisor offered the job to me. Of course, I accepted. The unit I was to run was an 18 bed unit with both detox patients and psychiatric patients. I had the experience and know-how to properly run the unit. I spent almost 4 ½ years as Manager. My staff was the best. They worked as an efficient team and I loved each and every one of them! I had the best of everything while I was in this position. My supervisors were totally supportive and there for me always. Even the Joint Commission on Accreditation of Health Organizations, JCAHO, was complimentary of our unit when they came to accredit our hospital. It was a great time.

I was well for some period of time. I even had my problems with minor illness, but I never let that stop me. My faith in God, Jesus Christ my Savior and His Beloved Blessed Mother have been there for me always. One thing I learned a long time ago was that any hard work done doesn't go unrecognized. Even today, while I write this book, I know that I will help some student out there' who needs that little encouragement to get by. Hang in there! You will make it if you work hard and apply what you have learned.

Not only was our move to Tennessee a successful one where work was concerned, but, I was ready to work on growing in my level of education. In 1999, I went back to school and eventually earned my Bachelor's Degree in Health Arts. This program was a bridge program for nurses who wanted to go on for their Master's Degree. At the time I graduated, I didn't think I wanted an advanced degree, but the more I thought about it, the more I said why not! I went back to school at The University of St. Francis in Joliet, Illinois, and pursued my Masters in Healthcare Administration. I managed to complete the program totally online. It wasn't difficult but the courses appeared to be easier than the undergraduate courses. (Perhaps too, it was because I was in the studying mode.) I managed to graduate with a 4.0 GPA in May of 2005. Later on, I will share with you my struggle to finish the last semester. I was 55 at the time.

Points to Ponder

1. Your life doesn't have to persecute you. It's like this....if you have a bunch of sour lemons, you can make lemonade from them. **Life is what you make it.** Life owes you nothing. God never said life would be easy, but He did say He would be there for you always. You just have to ask.

2. Follow your instincts when making decisions regarding your career or profession. If you don't take risks, you will never know what you may have become in life.

3. Follow a famous lady who once said to first put God in your life, family second and career third. She used this as her mission statement to run her company which continues to be successful today.

4. When you have personal issues, it's best to work on them by getting professional help. Not only did I get help for my co-dependency, but I have been working in a field that will help me to stay focused and work with my patients more efficiently and effectively.

5. Healthcare is constantly re-establishing itself. There are changes taking place on a daily basis. If you plan on staying in the "game," you must re-establish yourself. It may be taking on extra classes or going on for that degree. You MUST work on yourself and your resume' if you want to get ahead in life and your profession.

6. Those of you with families can start out with an Associates Degree in Nursing and after graduation,

pursue advanced degrees on a part-time basis. Unfortunately, unless you plan on advancing in your career as a manager or university instructor, most hospitals do not pay more in salary for **advanced degrees**.

7. Check with your employer for any information on tuition reimbursements. Many employers will pay a percentage of tuition and books if the degree earned will be an advantage or asset to their business. For example, a hospital may pay a percentage of Julie's tuition if she is pursuing a degree in Respiratory Therapy. The hospital may also ask for a period of time in service for the tuition paid. For example, Julie may receive the tuition for school and after graduation, spend the following 2 years in service to the hospital.

8. Nowadays, there are so many opportunities to go to school online. I completed my entire course for my Masters Degree online. It wasn't easy but, I was able to study at any time in my home. I could be up at midnight and get online to the school to complete a paper or get on the class chat room for discussion. It's really a great way to finish your course and earn a degree.

Chapter 4: Deadly Problems

The reason for writing this book has been in the back if my head a long time. Not long after a hospitalization that nearly killed me, I talked with the manager of the acute care where I was a patient. I had already returned to work as manager for my psych unit and thought about many things that occurred during my hospitalization that bothered me. I made a list of these items and gave them to the manager of the units so she could post them on a bulletin board in the break room for staff to read. The list was intended for the nurses caring for their unconscious patients. The more I thought about this, the more determined I was to write this book, hoping it would give them some insight and change their perceptions on patient care. I've written primarily background information so that readers could delve into the words and imagine in their minds the person I have been and continue to be. Life doesn't go on without growth. Everything I have experienced, whether good or bad, has made me a better person spiritually and emotionally. My body may be weak and crippled, but my heart is strong and my spirit everlasting. So, here it goes..........

I was returning to work as a manager for the psych unit after spending a week off during the holidays. I always set aside time to spend with my daughter and grandson at Christmas. My daughter is a nurse too and had to put in her time at work during the holidays. We usually worked every other Christmas. At this point in our lives, it didn't matter whether or not we were off Christmas day. We were just happy to be together. I didn't feel very good the morning I returned to work. The drive was 18 miles one way and I usually listened to my favorite radio station on the way to kill the monotony. I was only a few blocks away from the hospital when I developed respiratory problems. I became short of breath and parked quickly so I could get inside. I finally got to the door and headed for the Emergency Room. They registered me right away and before I knew it, I had an oxygen mask over my face. My O2 SATS were in the 80's and I was getting very anxious. I told the doctor several times that I needed a stress dose of steroids because of my Addison's Disease. I received 125 mg IV of Cortef which would prevent me from going into a crisis. I was eventually sent up to a room with the diagnosis of :an asthma attack with respiratory infection. All of this took place on a Monday. Little did I know I would be facing much more challenging problems. During that week, I received respiratory treatments around the clock. I was given IV antibiotics. My arms were bruised all over because the nurses had a difficult time trying to get the IVs in. I have small, deep veins. I received large doses of steroids during that week which helped the asthma and infection. I did well until waking up that Friday morning. I realized I had a mild pain in my lower right abdomen. The pain wasn't intense. It wasn't gas because gas moves around. I just couldn't pin point it. In fact, at one point, I wasn't going to even report it, but I did anyway. The doctor ordered a CT scan and the results were: PERFORATED DIVERTICULUM. OH MY GOD! What next? I've had problems in the past with my bowel/colon and figured this may not be too bad. The attending doctor called in a surgeon who felt that I was a high risk for surgery and that antibiotic therapy may be the best course to take. One of his partners, a very outspoken woman, stepped right in and said, "anyone who has a hole in their bowel has poop leaking through into the abdomen and it isn't good!" I asked her what she would do and she went to explain that I would have surgery with a colostomy; be on a ventilator in one of the units. That was a lot to swallow, let me tell you! She scheduled me for surgery the next morning on a cold Saturday. My family was there including my husband, Gail, daughter, Annette and son-in-law, Wayne. My grandson was being watched at home, but I wanted to see him so desperately. You can imagine how frightened I was about the whole process I was about to face. I prepared myself spiritually by seeing a priest for confession and communion and placed my scapular over my gown, asking the surgical staff not to remove it. I was ready to meet my Maker should this be my time. I kissed everyone I dearly loved at my bedside and off I went to the surgical waiting area. It was my understanding that the surgery took approximately 10 hours that day.

I was later told that I went into atelectasis during surgery. I developed Scleroderma as well. The doctor performed 5 surgeries in a matter of a few days. When she initially opened my abdominal cavity, she found I was already full of infection. Evidently, the steroids I had been receiving all week for my asthma camouflaged any signs of infection I may have been having. If you remember, I had very little pain and when they took my vital signs, I wasn't even running a fever. Now, the doctor had to irrigate my abdomen and work on the section of the bowel that had the perforated diverticulum. She put in place a colostomy which was revised 3 times before it would work properly. Once she had completed the series of irrigations, a wound vac was placed over the huge hole in my abdomen so that I could heal from the inside out. I wasn't aware of anything at the time because I was on a ventilator, maintained at an unconscious level. I also had a tracheostomy which maintained my airway. The nurses in the unit knew me because at one time, I was their supervisor. They would take turns caring for me. There were familiar faces to see once I was off the vent. In the meantime, my visitors were a bit overwhelming for me, so the doctor decided to limit visitors for awhile. A good friend of mine made a binder notebook for visitors to sign and write notes. At discharge, I took home a notebook full of notes from many friends and loved ones, but it took me 6 months to get the strength to open that book and read what they had to say. Needless to say, I was very touched by words of hope and love.

Occasionally, I will open that notebook and remind myself how precious life is especially when you have family and friends that love you. That's what life is all about!

I need to talk about what it's like to be a patient in an acute care unit, on a ventilator. I didn't feel any pain during my entire ordeal. I felt comfortable in spite of all the wires, tubes and IVs. I was in a bed that filled with air as I moved so that my body was supported all over. The ventilator had whistles and horns that I heard even while sedated. A person loses all sense of time while sedated. I couldn't tell the difference between one day and one week. One particular instant had me so upset believing I had been unconscious for years. During periods when my family was at my bedside, the nursing staff would allow me to waken just enough to realize my family was present. One nurse held up my grandson's picture and continued to say, "wake up Marilyn and look at your grandson's picture." I couldn't see because I didn't have on my glasses. I was lightly sedated and didn't realize where I was or what happened. I was being given Versed, a powerful drug that works to sedate and forget. The drug is stored in the fatty tissue of the body and takes a long time to be eliminated. I had this idea in my head that I was somewhere, but didn't know where! My daughter told me much later that when she came in to visit, she would tell me what my cardiac monitor showed, what my blood work was an how I was doing in general. The problem was I was forgetting as fast as I was being told information. *I thought I had lost years of time in a sedated state.* While sedated, I had these crazy dreams. One in particular is about me going to a Mexican restaurant. I was climbing rod-iron spiral steps and found at the top a large parrot, spitting out peanut shells in my face. After much thought, I realized later a nurse must have been washing my face. I dreamt of driving along a shoreline on the East coast and wanting to get out and walk along the sand. At that point in my dream, I was probably being given a bath. I remember at some point while sedated, someone spreading my legs and inserting something. I had this crazy dream of a nurse swinging from a trapeze and inserting a suppository up my vagina with her bare feet! I had developed a terrible vaginal yeast infection that spread to my inner thighs. The infection developed as a result of the massive antibiotic therapy I was receiving for the infection. My daughter, who is an RN, thought about my past experiences with antibiotics and told the doctor. The doctor, in turn, examined me to find this terrible yeast problem. I was only aware of the discomfort from the yeast infection when the nurses spread my legs to insert the suppository medication which burned and itched. It was then I had the vision of the nurse on the trapeze!

There were times I was just barely awake to see the room dark and I was thinking I was in my bedroom at home and someone was having a party in my backyard. I evidently attempted to climb out of the bed when the nurse walked in to stop me.

Dreams, to most people, are a part of our sleep process. Dreams experienced as a part of sedation can be very vivid. As I explained earlier, I had some really crazy dreams during sedation.

With all that was going on, never did I receive any sign that I was going to die. One of my sisters asked if I saw that "bright light people see when they're dying?" I told her no, because I wasn't dying! Often, I saw the face of Jesus in my sleep. As long as I saw His face, I was at peace. I could also pray during this time. I remember saying the Lord's prayer and Hail Marys many times while sedated. I would often ask myself what is going on. I would then ask Jesus what was going on, but didn't get an answer at that time.

One thing that I must bring up is being able to hear during sedation. It's important to remember that while a person is under sedation, he/she can still hear very clearly. I could hear my doctors discussing my problems, talking to staff. I do remember some of the nurses talking to me while they performed my care. Tone of voice is everything though. My husband came to visit one of many times. He stood at my bedside and one of the nurses lightened my sedation so that I could interact with him. My husband spoke to me with a trembling voice. In all the years of our marriage, did I ever hear his voice sound so troubled. Months later, I explained to him how upset I was to hear his voice like that. I understood he was upset too, but his voice frightened me. My daughter told me how often she held my hand and talked to me, telling me about Garrett, our grandson. I would squeeze her hand, letting her know I understood. But, remember, I was receiving drugs that made me forget. I was forgetting minute after minute. It was important that everyone around me repeat themselves, constantly reorienting me to date, time, place and how long I was there.

Over a period of 6 weeks, I remained in CCU before I was weaned from the ventilator. From a WBC of > 40,000, and in sepsis, I was brought back to a more normal condition when the doctors felt they could release me from the vent. The next chapter will discuss my weaning from the vent along with getting back to the job of living and adjusting. Please follow closely the Points to Ponder in this chapter. A patient's stay in a hospital can be made so much more comfortable, less painful and worrisome if you include them in your nursing practice. There is one other situation I don't want to forget and that is checking on your patient *frequently*. At one point while still being weaned from the ventilator, I was in a very physically uncomfortable position in my bed. I needed reposition-ing, turned and just as I call it, "fluffed, puffed and buffed!"

I hadn't seen a nurse in what I felt was a long time, (again, this has everything to do with the perception of the patient) and I grew more and more frustrated to the point of tears. There were several extra pillows on my bed which I was able to grasp and so I threw them out as far as I could onto the floor outside of my cubicle. To my amazement, staff of all different levels walked around those pillows, not stopping to pick them up, not stopping to see where they came from and above everything else, not stopping to check on me! Eventually, my nurse did come in and attend to me.

This may sound petty, but I couldn't believe it! For Pete's sake, if you see anything *unusual,* check it out.

Points to Ponder

1. Get involved in the post-operative care of the patient. Do not be afraid to examine wounds, dressings, special equipment. Learn how to operate special equipment in order to be comfortable with it. Ask another nurse to assist you in working with new equipment.

2. Practice listening to abdominal sounds using a CD purchased at your school or a company like Amazon.com. Using your stethoscope, listen to all 4 quadrants and identify any changes or sounds different from the norm.

3. Listen to your patients. Anxiety can be a symptom of decreased oxygen saturation. At this point, it would be a good idea to check the oxygen saturation of the patient.

4. If policy allows, use Lidocaine in prepping an IV site for catheter insertion, especially in those patients who are difficult to stick. It saves the patient a lot of discomfort.

5. Remember that there is usually more than one option in handling a crisis. Evaluate all aspects of situations before making a final decision.

6. Allow your patient time to vent his/her feelings upon learning of a serious situation or what they may have to face. This helps in lessening their anxiety level. Offer prescribed medication to assist them in resting.

7. "Listening" is sometimes all a patient wants of you without unsolicited advice.

DON'T YANK MY FOLEY!

8. Assist the patient in preparing physically and emotionally for their procedure, surgery, etc. by explaining each step in the process, in a clear and concise manner.

9. Include family in planning—they are concerned too and want to be a part of the process.

10. Ask the patient if they wish spiritual support from their pastor, priest or rabbi.

11. Visitors can wear down the patient's strength. Although they are welcome, the visitors need to be reminded when it's time to leave.

12. When working with professionals as patients, do not assume they know what is going on. Keep in mind the person is a **patient** at that moment. When it comes to healthcare professionals, we are a very dynamic breed of individuals who, in most cases, had numerous and varied experiences. I am sure there are nurses out there who don't know the meaning of MRSA!
Remember what the word **ASSUME** means?

13. A patient's perception of his/her surroundings can be very distorted at times. He/she is dealing with physical and emotional trauma, pain and worry about prognosis, finances and how his/her family will react to their situation.

14. No 2 patients are alike! Each reacts, responds, perceives, absorbs and listens in their own way based on their own personal coping skills or, lack of.

15. No 2 patients react to pain the same. You must respond to their requests for pain relief based on what they tell you using the pain scale from 0-10. Keep in mind that the patient may be laughing with a room full of visitors and yet be in pain. The patient is merely being distracted.

16. You may have to repeat yourself several times before the patient grasps onto the information.
Medications and the condition of the patient in general can affect how the patient retains information, therefore, it will be up to you to check with the patient often when giving directions and explanations.

17. Last but not least, ORIENT the patient frequently. Every time you enter the patient's room, remind them of what day it is, the time, and how many days they have been in the hospital. It is so easy to get disoriented when routine has been the case. Hours become days, days become weeks and more. Don't ever assume the patient remembers or understands. It is an idea to have the patient repeat what you said to determine his level of understanding.

18. Use all of your senses when assessing the patient. I am talking about eyes, ears, nose, smell. Your senses are God's gifts to you and they can be very useful in determining any problems the patient isn't able to point out.

19. It's very busy on the floor or in a doctor's office or making visits to your home care patients. Make sure you let the patient know when you are returning to the room, especially when the patient is frightened and worried. It will lessen the frequency of the call light ringing out if you

do. In the best of circumstances, patients are anxious, frightened, scared, angry, and do not need to be left in the dark regarding their care. Just by saying, "Mrs. Jones, I'm leaving now. Is there anything you need at this time? If not, I will be back in 30 minutes to check on you."

Chapter 5: Don't Yank My Foley

I finally get to the title of my book and you are probably wondering why I would use such a title. It all goes back to the early part of my story when I was being prepared for surgery on my colon. Most surgical nurses, or any floor nurse for that matter knows that insertion of a foley catheter is essential in keeping the patient comfortable, maintaining Intake and Output and preventing skin breakdown. I was going to have this huge colon surgery, be put in the Unit on a ventilator with very little chance of movement while maintained in an unconscious level. This was the best way to do all what the foley was intended to do. In the last chapter, I mentioned being in the CCU for 6 weeks while on the ventilator. The weaning process was done in steps and, what I might add as frightful to say the least. The tracheostomy was to be removed with an opened hole left in my neck to heal on its own. To my own surprise, I managed to overcome the fear and eventually was weaned from the trach. The next step was getting Physical Therapy involved in helping me to reach maximum mobility. They first started with my hands and arms because at this point, I was barely able to raise my hands off the bed. Therapy advanced to getting me to dangle at the side of the bed and eventually stand, using a walker. Now, getting back to my foley catheter; any nurse will tell you this is a little gadget consisting of a tube attached to an enclosed bag. The process of insertion is done by sterile technique. The nurse dons sterile gloves, and, after cleansing the meatus (on a woman, it's directly below the clitoris and above the vaginal opening) inserts the catheter beyond the meatus, up through the ureter until a stream of urine is seen flowing through the tube down into the bag. At this point, the catheter is pushed up a little more until its tip has reached just beyond the bladder entrance. The nurse will then insert a small amount of sterile water through a side vent taking the water to the tip of the catheter, inflating the tip so as to hold the catheter in place while draining the bladder. You are probably wondering "why in the world did she stop what she was saying to describe this foley?" I wanted you to understand just how very sensitive the area is where the foley catheter is located. When I mentioned dangling at the side of the bed for PT, my foley catheter was right there, dangling right alongside of me.

These catheters are funny things. They are what I call "necessary evils." Yes, they are important in maintaining I&O, maintain skin integrity and can give any healthcare worker an idea of what condition the patient is in, but, they can also be a royal menace! To explain what I mean, let me go on further in my story. Each day, Physical Therapy was in my room, energetic and ready to drag me out of my bed to get me started. No sooner did they have me on my feet, than one of them grabbed my foley, and with its hook, attached the foley bag to his belt! Not only did the movement yank the catheter, but, it also yanked my you-know-what! OUCH! DON'T DO THAT! After several apologies, the catheter was off the therapist's belt and hanging from the rim of the bed. It took me a good hour to compose myself after that ordeal.

Several times before, a similar incident occurred. While weaning off the ventilator, the staff would transfer me to a type of stretcher called a "Cardio Bed." Once they had me on the stretcher, it could be put into a sitting position without having to move me. The only problem was the transfer from my bed to the chair while it was in a stretcher position. Several CNAs (Certified Nursing Assistants) would position themselves at both sides of me, **YANK** my foley catheter and plop the tubing and bag on top of my legs as they proceeded to transfer me. Again, OUCH! DON'T DO THAT! Every time I was moved from one side to the other, the foley was *yanked* and pulled as well.

Every time I was pulled up in the bed, the foley was *yanked* and pulled as well. Also, holding the foley bag above the level of the patient's bladder will cause the urine in the bag to back-up into the bladder causing risk for infection. Continuous yank of the tubing against the sphincter muscles of the bladder, can weaken those muscles causing stress incontinence as well. It didn't take long for the staff to get the message when they handled my foley catheter inappropriately. The day that catheter was removed was the ultimate part of my hospitalization! I was a free woman, no longer tied down to a tube and "pee" bag. You know, when a woman says "DON'T YANK MY FOLEY!"...she means it! To this day, I feel every nursing staff member should have the experience of a catheter insertion and carry the entire contraption with them wherever they go. Perhaps a taste of their own medicine would do the trick in distinguishing the perils of a bedridden patient with the cursed FOLEY CATHETER!

Two weeks after weaning me off the trach, I was facing the possibility of going home after an asthma attack, through bowel surgery, recovery post-operatively and colostomy adjustment. The next chapter describes my introduction to a colostomy. During this period of recuperation, I gradually gained strength, performing my daily rounds around the floor where I was a patient. With my air-conditioned gown on, my no-skid socks, IV pole in one hand and wound vac in the other, I was pushed forward daily. I was in my final semester of grad school. I had maintained 4.0 GPA and just didn't want to go on any further in stalling the completion of my degree. My office was located around the corner from the unit I was on as a patient. Late at night around 11 PM, the nurses on the floor gave me the "go ahead" and let me walk down to my office to complete my school work online. For several weeks, I would sneak down to my office, work on my classes as I was hooked up to an IV and wound vac to my belly. I managed to finish my classes and eventually graduated in May, 2005 with a GPA of 4.0. My degree? Oh yes, Masters of Science in Health Services Administration.

Points to Ponder

1. Provide plenty of privacy when performing any intrusive procedure. Be empathetic to the feelings of the patient and their modesty. When acquiring the equipment, be mindful of the different types of sizes of catheters. The diameter of the catheter makes a big difference in comfort level for the patient. Most nurses use a #16 French but, honestly, if you can use a #14, it's a lot more comfortable. Take my word for it. I've been through this more than once.

2. Before insertion of a foley catheter, explain its purpose, the importance of maintaining sterility, proper positioning in relation to the bladder.

DON'T YANK MY FOLEY!

3. Never hang the foley bag on the bedside rail where it could be raised. Hang the bag only on the rim of the bed.

4. Monitor color and consistency of urine in the bag for any changes in the patient's condition.

5. Listen to the patient if they complain of spasms, burning, feelings of wanting to urinate and report symptoms to attending doctor.

6. Monitor other staffs' handling of patient's catheter, reminding them of proper positioning and handling.

7. Measure urine and empty foley bag regularly; preferably every shift.

8. Provide peri care to the patient on a regular basis, preferably daily to prevent infection.

9. Perform peri care at the foley site frequently, preferably daily. Watch for any signs of skin breakdown.

10. Unless contraindicated, encourage the patient to drink plenty of water in order to keep the foley flushed well.

Chapter 6: Adjusting to a Colostomy

The day before surgery on my colon, I was informed I would be receiving a colostomy. I didn't react strongly to this news because, as I figured it, I was a nurse; I could handle this and, I worked with colostomies many times over the years. After the initial surgery, the surgeon had to revise the colostomy 2 more times before it would function properly. The ostomy/wound care nurse came daily to check the colostomy and change the ostomy pouch. I was too sick at the time to even look at it so, a good month went by before I had the strength to sit up and examine it.

Upon returning home after 2 ½ months of hospitalization, I was very happy to see the familiar walls of my bedroom. Having no training whatsoever except the few crash instructions I gave him, my dear, sweet husband took on the task of cleaning the stoma and changing the pouch daily until I was strong enough to handle it myself. Not only that, but at no time, did I contract an infection by his handling of the surgical wound site and stoma care. To this day, I owe my husband, Gail, much love and gratitude for all he did.

My colostomy is actually flush to the skin, located in the crease on the left side of my mid-abdomen. Because of its position, we initially had a terrible time finding a pouch that would stay on.

After much trial and error with the help of a local ostomy/wound care shop, we were able to find a one-piece ostomy pouch I could wear in comfort along with a special adhesive attachment that would secure the pouch to my skin for at least 24-48 hrs. For the first few weeks when I took on the task for myself, I was a bit overwhelmed. The stoma is a deep, beefy-red area which is actually part of the colon that was brought to the surface and secured in place. I have no control of my bowel movements and watch the amount of fiber or lack of, I eat. If I don't monitor my food intake, I can have a terrible time with constipation or diarrhea. I had a lot of feelings about going to bed at night wearing a pretty gown and being close to my husband. I knew he loved me; there was no doubt about that. But, I felt very self-conscious about it along with the possibility of odor. I was using a special deodorant product I inserted inside the pouch, but even then, I was very self-conscious about the situation. It has taken me several years to adjust to the presence of the colostomy, even when my husband says he doesn't realize it's there most of the time. As far as he's concerned, I make the big deal out of it, not him. He hasn't as yet to this day shown any signs of disgust towards me or my colostomy. In some respect, I put myself in the same position as a woman who has had a breast mastectomy.

It has been 5 years since I received the colostomy. I have adjusted to it and it doesn't bother me near as much. As for now, the colostomy is an everyday part of my routine of cleaning and grooming. I have found better and less expensive products to use such as pouches, sprays and stomahesive powder to use if the skin gets excoriated around the stoma. While working in the hospital, I have offered my time visiting patients who have fresh colostomies so they can see one can live a normal and

DON'T YANK MY FOLEY!

healthy life with it. As far as I'm concerned, my life (and love life) have not been impeded upon by the colostomy, AND, above everything else, it's a **small price to pay for maintaining my life.**

The next and final chapter basically summarizes all that happened those 5 years ago. With it, are points to ponder and apply as those of you continue in your nursing profession. I learned long ago, you are never too old to learn something new.

Points to Ponder

1 If a patient happens to be on the unit, ask them to look at their colostomy if you haven't seen one.

2. Get acquainted with the different types of stomas of patients, the location of the stomas in relation to the patient's body. Location determines what part of the bowel is affected and the type of-output it will produce.

3. Encourage a patient with a new colostomy to look at, examine it and know to recognize its normal features.

4. Give the patient time to vent and share his/her feelings regarding the colostomy. Don't push them into looking at it if they don't want to.

5. Encourage the patient to share concerns regarding odor and intimacy with their partner. Let them know there are many good products on the market for discreetness

6. Encourage family members, spouses or partners to take part in the care of the stoma. Allow them to vent their concerns and feelings. Encourage them to reassure the patient of their feelings for him/her during the adjustment period.

7. Introduce the patient to other patients or staff, if possible who also have colostomies.

8. Obtain a list of suppliers in the area where the patient can go for more support and information in caring for their colostomy.

9. Remind the patient that adjustment takes time. No 2 patients are alike. Tell them to allow 6 months to a year to feel comfortable with their colostomy

10. If the surgeon told the patient the colostomy could be reversed, remind the patient to keep that in mind. For those of you who are nurses, the patient has to come to the realization that he/she will have to be the one to take care of the colostomy. A spouse or family member may help in the beginning but, essentially, the patient will have to come to grips with it and work with it. BUT, it all comes in time.

Chapter 7: Peace and Acceptance

Five years seems like such a long time ago, but what I described in these chapters remain with me as clear as if it all happened yesterday. Although I faced death in the face, I would experience it all over again because of how it changed me as a person. When one is as sick as I was, you're never the same. So many doctors, nurses, my husband, daughter and friends were there by my side, supporting me; loving me for me! I can never forget that. Illness is a terrible thing, but it made me stronger as a person, a Christian and fellow human being. I can never repay those who helped me through those terrible months as I lay in a hospital bed, on a ventilator, barely making it from day to day. The knowledge, technology, hours of loyalty and commitment all played a part in my "success" story . I am so proud to be a part of that winning team of healthcare workers who face different challenges everyday so that people like myself, can experience that second chance at quality life.

Epilogue

Since March of this year (2009), I have had some unexpected health issues that placed me back in the hospital. From a colonoscopy to back surgery with complications, I still have not given up in the wonderful profession of Nursing I feel so proud to be a part of today. Yes, there are those of you just getting started on your careers with a few years already notched on your belts. To you, I raise my hands and applaud your tenacity. You are the foundation of Nursing as it is today and will be in the future. To those of you who have been in "the field" for quite some time, I bow to you for your strength of wisdom, patience, perseverance and "power to the people" attitude. Combined, all of you confirm my hope in the continuance of Nursing as a respected and dignified profession, demanding the attention and honor it so rightfully deserves.

My experiences as a patient the past months have been for the most part, great! I have met some wonderful people who took part in my care. I do want to comment on a couple of people who stood out from the bunch. You know who you are, and yes, take credit where credit is due. One nurse in particular was above all else, sublime. She didn't stay on the unit but a short time, transferring to a unit who would no doubt benefit from her skills the moment she arrived. This person was warm, sensitive and very intuitive. She possessed the **HEART OF A MODEL NURSE**. She made my concerns, hers. She made my moments of pain, anger and frustration, hers. Every time she walked down the hall, her entire demeanor was that of professionalism. Before discharge, I had the opportunity of speaking to this nurse's manager. The manager felt she was losing someone very special, but realized it didn't matter where this nurse went; any patient was going to benefit from the care she delivered.

What was so great about my experience with this person was my responses to her!

I looked forward to her coming on duty. I looked forward to seeing her warm smile. I **FELT** better physically and emotionally **BECAUSE** of her empathy, sense of humor, honesty and attention to my needs. I took away from this experience a sense of well-being and hope for my future needs as a patient if and when the time comes.

The other nurse I want to mention cared for me 2 nights in a row. He was a gentleman of my age and mentioned being a nurse 20 years. What was so interesting about him was his accomplishments in life and how he came to nursing. We were able to share our views on the dynamics of nursing and how changes in healthcare have turned caring into a big-business. Unfortunately, he didn't have much time to talk. I admired his focus to detail and although he was moving at a fast pace, he was able to discuss with me my medical condition as it was at that moment, completing his assessment in a timely manner and administering my medications. He was warm, smiled a lot and just easy to talk to about my concerns. This nurse, although male, offered a female nurse come in should I feel uncomfortable about my privacy. I declined. Basically, he thought of *everything* to help me feel comfortable with him as my care giver. Again, professionalism was what I saw in this man.

DON'T YANK MY FOLEY!

To those nurses out there contemplating leaving Nursing or a particular area of Nursing, if this is what you need for yourself, by all means, ***DO IT!*** As much as I have loved Nursing, there is a point in all of our careers when enough is enough and we need out. My philosophy is when Nursing no longer provides for you the sense of pride in helping others; no longer gives you a feeling of a job well done, then it is time to make some major decisions. I saw this too, during my recent hospital stays. Sure, we all have our bad days on the job when nothing seems to go right. That, in itself, is life. ***How*** we pick ourselves up is the key. When a nurse flies into a patient's room, stating the floor is short-staffed, complaining about a patient in the next room, complaining about personal issues at home, a patient gets the feeling he/she is in the way and will hold back when it comes to voicing their needs. ***I found myself doing that, and frankly, no patient wants to hear that from their care-givers.*** If you find yourself as a nurse, displaying these behaviors in a regular manner, it's time to get out and do some self-re-evaluation. Let me tell you, no patient wants to be "short-sheeted" verbally, physically and emotionally. They don't need it, and frankly, you don't need it. You end up selling yourself short as a nurse, a professional and fellow human being. If you are at this point it is best to just get out.

Points to Ponder

1. Remember who you are as a person and a nurse.

2. Treat every human being as special and individual.

3. Return to this book periodically to "freshen" your views and perceptions on patient care.

4. It's good to make shortcuts in nursing, *as long as it doesn't interfere in the quality of nursing care you give. If you do, you are shorting yourself as a nurse AND your patient!*

The End

CPSIA information can be obtained at www.ICGtesting.com
Printed in the USA
BVOW03s1453190114

342368BV00002B/153/P